Peculiar Habits of Extra-Ordinary
PEOPLE

D1607973

Peculiar Habits of Extra-Ordinary
PEOPLE

Patrick Lowe, D.C.

Dr. Lowe page (502) 245-7334
drlowe@lowechiro.com
or visit Patricklowe.com

This book was written the old fashioned way, without the use of AI. Special Thank you to my Editor Ricky Ricardo, BA .

Your Human Intelligence made this possible.

TABLE OF CONTENTS

INTRODUCTION

Have you ever noticed those people? The ones who don't seem to follow all the rules, they march to the beat of a different drum. I don't know when I started noticing them. I mean really noticing them. In a group of people they are scattered about, but somehow they stand out. They are happy, positive, healthy people. People feel attracted to and want to be around them and to engage in conversation. There is just something different about them.

They continue to do things long after most people their age have given them up. They keep riding horses, hopping on go carts, four wheelers, and working out. It's difficult to guess their age because they don't act it. Even worse, when they don't look their age either. They look much, much younger. These people remain healthy and able to do things long after their peers have been sidelined.

It's not plastic surgery or a magic pill. It's not a life of self-deprivation. It's not living in the gym.

Their habits are peculiar. That's what gives them an extra-ordinary life!

So, where do we begin?

I recently heard that the first person who will live to be 150 years old has already been born. Dr. Eric Plasker in his Book *The 100 Year Lifestyle* points out that The number of people who are living to be over 100 yrs old is growing every year. Which means that you have a better chance now, than any other time in history to live into your 100 and beyond.

Whether you have one year left or 150 years to look forward to, one question is the same. How do you want to live those years?

As we ponder over that question it is important for us to make a distinction between the words "average" and "Extra-Ordinary"

AVERAGE VS EXTRA-ORDINARY
Average

Average is a *mathematical term*. To figure the average you take a group of numbers, add them up and divide by the number of numbers. Some numbers will be higher, some lower but the average of the group of numbers is somewhere in the middle. Our brains do that with our environment. If everyone around us has, bad teeth, we expect that we will also have bad teeth, but if a great dentist comes to town and teaches you how to brush, floss, and get regular check ups, you improve your odds at surpassing the average.

Habits of the Average:

Average people wait for a crisis before they consider making changes. "If it ain't broke, don't fix it" or "If it doesn't hurt, leave it alone." is the mindset. The whole time, they are degenerating in so many ways.

One patient, a runner, who looked at me and said "Doc, I plan to wear out, not rust out!"

He was 65 and always looking for ways to stay healthy and active. Now he was *Extra-Ordinary*

The average person may even stay active, but still wait in until pain strikes before they make changes. Then they resort to some sort of crisis care. They look for help only when they are in severe pain, broken down or unable to do their normal routines. Then when the perceived crisis is over… they go back to doing everything that caused the crisis in the first place, until the next crisis occurs. Even so, there are a lot of people who try to live better lives, but the advice they follow leaves out the most important things.

People who live average lives, get average results. They feel worse than they could. They miss out on more than they should, and they settle for a mediocre life. This is because they just don't know that there are any other ways to do life.

When they become aware of other ways to live, they don't believe that it's possible for them. Although, once they know it's possible, they don't know how to change their habits to the life they really want.

EXTRA-ORDINARY HUMANS

Extra-ordinary is something that stands above what is average; it is in a category all its own. I don't know about you but I have never wanted to just be average or just normal; nor do I want to be average in my income, my health, my happiness or my abilities. Children practice a sport with dreams of being Extra-ordinary! They dream of making the game winning pass in the Super Bowl, the final pitch in the World Series, or of winning a Gold medal in the olympics. They want to surpass all expectations. This sort of aspiration shouldn't just be limited to the sports we play as kids; it should also extend to other areas of life.

If you do what everyone else does, you will get what everyone else gets. Extra-ordinary people don't just follow the pack.

In our lives, our health and our longevity, we want to take it a step further. We want to go beyond standard expectations. We want to be Extra-ordinary.

The following chapters will tell you what the Extra-ordinary humans do to become that way.

So what do Extra-ordinary humans have in common? On the surface, not much, but when you dig deeper, they reveal some telling habits and they have principles & secrets that you can copy and paste into your life to make a huge impact on your present and your future.

One of the secrets is that they automate the principals that we will be discussing. These principles are their habits and lifestyles. Setting yourself up for success requires a deep understanding of habits.

Once we understand how to make real change, we can stop grinding through new things hoping that it will, somehow… against our will… become a lifelong habit.

One of the peculiar habits of the Extra-Ordinary is that they prioritize things differently.Some have developed these priorities on their own by doing their own research and changing their habits. Others were just more naturally inclined to prioritize their life this way. Then there is a third group who were taught these peculiar habits by their friends and loved ones.

In the next 2 hours we will unpack the secrets of the Extra-ordinary.

Here's to living an Extra-ordinaryLife!

COMMAND CENTER
PRIORITY 1

I

I used to do a weekly new patient class and invite all of our patients and their friends to come hear about how to maximize their health.

I ask my classes to prioritize these systems of the body. And number them from most important to least important; #1 being most important and #4 being least important.

___ The cardiovascular system with the heart and lungs

___ The digestive system

___ The nervous system

___ The endocrine system which produces hormones

What do you think?

A lot of people say the Cardiovascular system is most important.

One particular Wednesday night, no patients showed up, just one guy. His name was Jake. Jake was in college and looking at a career in medicine. He was curious about what we did, as chiropractors.

I started the presentation and asked Jake the same question I ask everyone:

Doc: "Which system of the body is the most important?"

Jake: "You know, When you are having a heart attack, not much else matters."

Doc: "Yes, you're right"

Doc: "However, Do you know how long you can live without food?"

He shrugged

Jake: "More than 40 days."

Doc "How about water?"

Jake:"A day?" he guessed

Doc: "About 4 days. Now how about air?"

Jake: He smiled. "They say about 4 minutes before it starts causing brain damage."

Doc: "You're right."

I paused for a moment and then I asked him this:

Doc: "What does lack of food, lack of water, lack of air do to the body?"

Jake: "It will cause brain damage."

Doc: "So how long can you live without brain waves?"

Jake: "Ohhhhh…." I saw the light go on, as he got it.

Jake: "How long can you live without brain waves?"

Now this was the question that really put it into perspective. So I answered him.

Doc: "Maybe 4 seconds… We don't really know. We know that we can't restart the brain, like they do a heart after bypass surgery. Once it stops, we are dead."

He was quiet for what felt like an eternity while I waited for him to come up with his next question. He stood up and walked over the chart on the wall that shows all of the nerves and where they go.

Jake: "The brain and nervous system are the most important. It controls every other part of the body. Why don't you hear much about it then?"

Doc: "Strange isn't it?"

Jake: "Tell me more…"

Doc: "What kind of movies do you like?" I asked, hoping he wouldn't say romantic comedies.

Jake: "Action movies"

Doc: "Have you ever noticed that they are always trying to destroy the command center or get to the top guy?"

Jake: "Yeah…"

Doc: "The battle is to defeat the mastermind or take over control of the *command center*. Small victories are made by disrupting communication."

Jake: "Okay?"

Doc: "Movie patrons intuitively understand the significance here. The control center is what guides the system and directs all defenses and the resources. The control center is also coordinating attacks against intruders. Without the control center the system cannot function. In the case of the body the control center is the brain and the nervous system."

Jake: "So our goal is to protect the brain and the nerves first?"

Doc: "Yes!" I was getting excited. This was the answer I was looking for.

Doc: "In the movies, where does the control center get its information and resources? From the intelligence in the environment, reports or cameras etc."

Jake: "Communication?"

Doc: "Yup, how does the body communicate with the brain?

Jake: "Through the nerves."

Doc: "Exactly. The primary goal of extra-ordinary people is to protect and preserve the control center and communication. All of the other systems of the body are designed to report to the brain and respond to its commands. The other systems also provide everything that the brain needs, oxygen, food, movement etc."

Jake: "I get it"

THE COMMAND CENTER AND COMMUNICATION:

So let me ask you what is more important; a healthy brain or a healthy body?

Well a sharp and active brain, if it is paired with a broken down, disabled body leads to frustration. It's frustrating when you lose your ability to do the things that you used to be able to do.

On the other hand an active body with a dysfunctional brain leads to frustration for others. Because we see either of these so frequently, it's often considered "Normal aging".

Actually both the brain and body are both very important. In the brain is your ability to think, feel and adapt; it regulates everything going on in your body. In the body is the ability to respond to the demands of the brain. I call that "Respond-ability" However, by order of priority, neurology comes first.

CASE STUDY: JEREMIAH

There's a young man named Jeremiah with quite the extra-ordinary story. His mom brought him to our office. He was 10 years old and he was having problems… a lot of problems. He had ADHD, problems with impulsivity, he didn't sleep and was causing a ton of stress for his adoptive family.

He was on the verge of being expelled from school and family life was tough.

They looked at sending him to boarding school and had been turned down 3 times.

He was taking so many medications including Vyvanse, Ritalin, Zoloft and a sleeping pill …… in adult dosages.

We got him under care, getting chiropractic adjustments on a regular basis. After 3 months we were seeing some progress. However, his mom needed a break, so she sent him with a friend to spend a couple of weeks away. After she had dropped him off, she realized that she had forgotten most of his medications at home.. 3 hours away.

She offered to mail them but the friend said she would take what she had and see how it goes.

Two weeks later, Jeremiah returned home. He walked in the door, sat down and started reading a book. When he was finished reading the book, he put his stuff away and started playing quietly.

When his mom saw this she thought to herself, "I couldn't believe what I was seeing." Then she looked over and told her friend, "You must be a better mom than I am."

However, her friend reassured her that that was not the case, and she reported that he had actually run out of meds after only 2 days. He had been like that since he ran out of meds.

His mom realized that something had changed, but had he 'grown out' of all of those problems in only two weeks or had the changes occurring in his body changed the processing in his brain?

We will unpack more about Jeremiah's story in following chapters.

Your brain controls every part of your body throughout your entire life.

Not only is your brain reading and interpreting this book, it is regulating your heart rate and your breathing. It's the natural pacemaker to your heart. It is signaling your stomach to digest the food that you last ate. If it's hot where you are, your brain is telling your skin to sweat. If it's cold, it is telling your muscles to shiver.

While all of this is going on, it is coordinating thousands of little muscle contractions in your feet, legs and core to keep you standing upright. It's doing everything from controlling balance and listening to your music.

In the event of a cut or injury, the nervous system directs local blood supply to increase and starts the inflammatory process. When the nerves have been damaged, normal healing does not occur. This is why people with diabetic neuropathy (damaged nerves) get cuts that don't heal etc.

All of this is controlled primarily by your brain and nervous system.

HOW DOES THIS WORK?

Impulses start in the brain and travel down through the spinal cord to give commands to the muscles, organs and tissues.

The body reports billions of bits of information back to the brain. Your brain prioritizes and interprets this information and responds.

The brain and spinal nerves have been mapped out and are being studied in great detail.

- The spinal nerves located in your upper neck are connected to the head and the face. They effect, headaches, dizziness, and blurred vision.
- The nerves in the lower and middle portions of your neck are connected to arms, hands, thyroid gland, and neck muscles.
- The nerves in your upper back communicate with the heart and lungs.

- The nerves in the middle part of your back take care of the valves around the stomach, the stomach, and small intestines.
- The nerves in your lower back go to the colon, uterus and ovaries in women and male reproductive organs in men. These nerves also are also connected to the muscles of your legs and feet.

When these pathways are open, the body can sense what's going on both inside and out. It can communicate this information to the brain and begin the most appropriate adaptation response.

When the pathway is closed or disrupted, either no information or incorrect information is sent to the brain. Without proper information the body will not adapt properly.

Again, a top priority for Extra-ordinary Humans is to keep their nervous system healthy and communicating with their bodies and their bodies communicating with the brains.

SUPPLY LINES
PRIORITY 2

II

Jake wanted to grab coffee. I was happy to meet him at a local coffee shop to continue our conversation. I was curious to see what questions he had come up with since our last talk.

After some small talk, I started to ask him a couple questions.

Doc: "So what's on your mind?'

Jake: "Well, I couldn't stop thinking about what we talked about."

Doc: "Which part?"

Jake: "All of it, but I feel it's missing something, like it's not the whole story."

Doc: "Hmm. What's missing then?"

Jake: "I get how the brain controls the body and communication to and from the body is most important, but that leaves a lot of stuff out."

When I heard this I started to prod at his thoughts.

Doc: "Like what?"

Jake: "Like..." he paused and pulled out a notebook. "What about other things we see all the time?"

He started reading of a list that said: Heart attacks?
Poor nutrition?
Bleeding to death?
Suffocation?

After hearing his lists I started to explain to him.

Doc: "They fall under back to the second and third priorities of Extra-Ordinary People."

Jake: "What are the second and third priorities?"

Doc: "The second priority refers to the **supply lines.** The third refers to the **supply depot.** How do heart attacks, poor nutrition, bleeding to death or suffocation cause someone to die?"

Jake: "They all deprive the brain of something that it needs like blood carrying oxygen and food."

Doc: "Right, going back to our movie example. If the bad guy can't get directly to the command center, they try to disrupt the supply lines of food and other supplies from getting to the troops. Or kind of like how when invaders lay siege to a city, they cut the city off from their sources of food, water and reinforcements. So the blood supply to the brain and the body is super important for maintaining health, because it *supplies the* oxygen, nutrients, and food to the brain and the body."

Jake: "Don't the brain and nerves control the blood flow?"

Doc: "Yes, they control the arteries and shunt oxygenated blood from one artery to another as needed. They cause the smooth muscles around some arteries to contract and make the artery smaller while relaxing the smooth muscle around another artery to allow more blood flow. Have you ever had cold hands or cold feet when it's warm outside?"

Jake: "Yes"

Doc: "The body is moving the blood from your hands and feet to other vital parts of the body that need it more."

Jake: "How can we keep that in good shape?"

Doc: "Well, there are three ways:

The first is to use the system. The veins and lymphs are passive by themselves, but movement of the big muscles around them act as an external pump."

Jake: "So you are saying exercise?"

Doc: "I like to refer to it as movement; the more the muscles move, the better things go."

Doc: **"The second way is controlling your state.** We are always in either a state of excitement/Stress, the Sympathetic state, or we are in a state of 'rest and digest', Parasympathetic state."

Doc: "These states are controlled by the nervous system, by the foods we eat, and the stress hormones we build up. The sympathetic state increases blood pressure when we need it and the parasympathetic state lowers our blood pressure and improves our moods."

Jake: "Another loop?"

Doc: "What do you mean?"

Jake: "The parasympathetic state allows us to rest and digest. But the foods we eat can increase our stress?."

Doc: "Yup, things like too much processed foods or sugar will increase the stress hormone cortisol which stimulates the stressed Sympathetic state."

Jake: "What are the keys to transitioning back to a restful state?"

Doc: **"Well it's your nervous system being in balance,** what you eat, what you think, how much you move, and your environment.

My patients come to me for chiropractic adjustments to balance their nervous system when it is needed. What you eat determines what nutrients go to your brain, body and nerves. How much you move helps the blood flow but also helps your heart and lungs function to bring in the oxygen and pump it around."

Doc: "The third way is deciding what you put into the system and when.

but that will have to wait until another time, I've got patients waiting."

Back to Jeremiah's story: His mom continued to bring him to our office for care. As he grew up, they both noticed that he did a lot better in school and in life when he got adjusted regularly. Could Chiropractic adjustments be balancing his brain and helping him function better?

We had seen this effect and heard reports for years about kids doing better in school and behaviorally when under chiropractic care. Recent research from Dr Stephanie Sullivan demonstrated that both complex Physical Therapy exercises and a Chiropractic adjustment stimulate the area of the brain called the cerebellum and the prefrontal cortex. However, one difference between the results of the two treatments was that after 24 hours the effects of the physical therapy exercises started to decline. In contrast to this the effects of the chiropractic adjustments continued to increase for an entire week. Furthermore, additional adjustments increased the positive effects even more.

Geek out time!

The receptors in the spine stimulate the cerebellum. The cerebellum is the back of the brain. It holds half of the neurons (nerve cells) in the brain. Scientists used to think it only played a role in balance and coordination. New research with modern imaging shows that it does a whole lot more. It also processes sensory information from the body and plays a role in emotions and decision making. It also communicates with the prefrontal cortex and stimulates it.

The prefrontal cortex plays a crucial role in executive functions such as decision making, planning, problem solving, working memory, and attention control. The PFC also plays a role in regulating emotions and social behavior, as well as in modulating the activity of other brain regions. In addition, the PFC is involved in self-awareness and conscious thought. It inhibits pain, mood, autonomics (like heart rate and blood pressure), and it inhibits flexors (the muscles on the front of the body that make us walk bent over)

Neurological researcher Dr. Heidi Haavik says in her book *The Reality Check* that the Chiropractic Adjustment is "a bit like rebooting a computer."

CASE STUDY PART 2:

Let's apply this to Jeremiah's case. He was getting chiropractic adjustments regularly, he was running cross country/track and exercised a lot. **Maintaining communication channels between the brain and the body is the primary focus of Chiropractic care. We work to correct interference between the body and the brain. If there is tension or pressure on the nervous system the communication breaks down.**

Both exercise and adjustments stimulate and balance the areas of the brain that process emotion, self awareness and social behaviors and attention control.

His behaviors improved as he could focus, process emotion and be more self aware. He could also interact with other people better.

He is an Extra-Ordinary human.

So while your brain controls your body, your body helps balance the brain.

In addition to chiropractic adjustments, there are the 3 M's of brain balancing:

Movement, Music, and Meditation.

- Movement: Just like complex physical therapy, movement stimulates the brain. Exercises that use both sides of the body also help as well. Exercises like walking, running, rowing, or just general workouts.

- Music: Functional MRI studies show that listening to music stimulates both sides of the brain. Playing a musical instrument or singing coordinates the entire brain.
- Meditation: Finally prayer and meditation help calm our brains and help us return to a more relaxed state.

I know this may sound contradictory, first I said stimulate the brain, then I said calm the brain. The reality is though that we need both in order to balance the brain, just like breathing in and breathing out. Too much breathing in and we will pass out, if we just breathe out we will also pass out. Just like the natural rhythm of breathing in and out; in and out is the key; stimulate the brain and calm the brain.

SUPPLY DEPOT
PRIORITY 3

III

Jake and I met up at our usual coffee shop and sure enough he paid. We got settled in at a table as he opened his trusty notebook.

Jake: "So where does nutrition and oxygen fit in?"

Doc "That fits into priority # 3"

Jake: "Why is that #3?"

Doc: "You can have all of the best oxygen and the best nutrition in the world, if it can't be sent to the right places in the right quantities when it is needed, it is useless."

Jake: "Huh?"

Doc: "We call this the Supply Depot. If a city is under attack and all of their food, medical supplies are in a supply depot 100 miles away and can't get to the city, it doesn't matter what is in that depot. It can't help them."

Jake: "How does that apply to people? We don't have huge stores of supplies in our bodies."

Doc: "You're right. A supply depot isn't about storage, it's about distribution. Storage on the other hand, happens in a warehouse. The depot is the connection between where things are brought in and sent back out. I think of it like a train depot, where things get loaded and unloaded here."

Doc: "For people, the supplies are the foods we eat, the air we breath and the water we drink. We want to fill our bodies with good things, break them down to usable parts and put them in the supply lines to get to wherever we need them.

In our bodies it's not a physical place that we store supplies. We operate like the Toyota car manufacturer. They don't have a big warehouse that holds parts for hundreds of cars. They manage their inventory so the parts arrive "Just-in-time" to make cars that week.

The human body is just like that. It doesn't store a lot of excess stuff. What it doesn't need, it secretes through the lungs, kidney or feces."

The parts arrive at the Toyota plant on big palates, all wrapped up. The parts are only usable when they are unwrapped and sent to the line to be put on cars.

Our nutrients come all wrapped up in our foods. Our bodies have to break them down and absorb them to actually become part of our usable supplies. Same with the air we breathe. We can take in all the air we want, *but if the lungs can't properly absorb the oxygen from it, it doesn't help our "Just in time" Supply depot.*

Jake: "But, how does fat fit into the equation?"

Doc: Hmm. Good question. We can overload the supply depot. When we do that, the body defaults to building extra storage at the supply depots for emergency food rations.

It is a survival strategy. So because of an overload of supply, what is originally only meant to be short term storage before distribution ends up becoming long term storage.

Like we talked about earlier, Extra-ordinary people move more and eat better than average people so there's a proper balance between incoming supplies and the use of those supplies. They regulate their "just in time" inventory by what they take in. They also work to put only good things into their bodies.

The supply depot is the third priority because we need communication and a properly functioning supply chain before we worry about what supplies have arrived at the depot."

Jake: "It sounds like they are teaching it all wrong in school."

Doc: "How so?"

Jake: "Health classes and science classes in schools talk a lot about eating right and exercising but that's as far as it goes."

Doc: "What do they mean by eating right?"

Jake: "Following the *MyPlate* portions of food, avoiding junk food, stuff like that."

Doc: "It's funny how that information changes. When I was a kid it was the 4 Food Groups, then it was the *Food Guide Pyramid*, then *MyPlate*. Why do you think they keep changing it?"

Jake: "I don't know, maybe because Americans are getting bigger and sicker all the time."

Doc: "Even with all the right foods, if the priorities are upside down people can't get the results they want."

Doc: "Do they talk about avoiding certain foods or food additives?"

Jake: "Sure, avoid processed foods, don't drink too many sodas, you know."

Doc: "Once we make sure the Command and Communication is in place, the supply lines are working, and the supply depot has the right stuff in it,

We have to avoid poisons and rats in the supply depot."

Jake: "Go on."

Doc: "Certain food additives and chemicals act like poison to our supply depot."

Jake: "Like a food allergy?"

Doc: "Right. For some people, then there are poisons that affect everyone. Things like glutamate, glyphosate and artificial sweeteners like aspartame. These are neurotoxins that damage the command center."

Jake: "You also said Rats? What are those?"

Doc "Rats steal the food and necessary nutrients from the supply depot. They give bad advice that makes us avoid good foods."

"In the 1980s the big push was to go fat free. The less fat people ate the fatter and sicker they became. We need good fats in our diets. The rats (the bad advice) made people afraid to eat what our bodies need."

Doc: "**Extra-ordinary work to eat better than the normal american diet.**

So Jake, do you know the difference between food and a poison?"

Jake: "I am not sure what you are getting at."

Doc: "At what dosage does aspirin become a poison."

Jake: "I don't know, I know to call poison control if someone takes a lot of any medicine."

Doc: "Great, the difference between a medicine and a poison is dosage.

The same is true for foods. Too much of a 'good thing' can be bad."

Jake: "You mean like vitamins?"

Doc "Yes. I mean like food in general, certain vitamins, certain minerals. There are a lot of things for the body to try to balance out. Too much of anything can be a bad thing."

Jake: "Even coffee"

We both laughed

Doc: "Jake, I have to get back to my patients."

Jake: "Let's grab coffee next week."

Doc: "Deal, but I have some homework for you. Do some research on the definition of Health. Try to figure out, what does it mean to be healthy?"

Jake: "You got it."

CASE STUDY PART 3:

Jeremiah's mom was recognizing amazing results in her son and her entire family. He was off of all of his prescribed medication. She asked me what supplements he should be taking. He was feeling anxious, his sleep was better but not great.

We decided to start him on coconut oil as a supplement. My thought process was that he was depleted of some essential fatty acids from his early years of poor nutrition.

I knew our brains require a lot of fats.

Essentially, we were trying to get things to his supply depot.

She started him immediately with some capsules from the local health food store.

The school had noticed his improvements as well.

The school's policy prevented him from taking coconut oil capsules without a prescription from a medical provider. That well intended policy was a Rat for Jeremiah.

His mom was smart and made him a whole food chocolate treat with organic coconut oil that he could eat during school.

We noticed that his anxiety in school continued to improve with his snacks and so did his concentration.

Jeremiah's mom kept him under chiropractic care to balance his nervous system, she kept him on coconut oil to feed his brain with essential fats, and she kept him on track so he could move and get lots of exercise. All the while she continued to be a very involved mom, helping him learn life's lessons and frequently used exercise as part of his discipline.

Stocking the supply depot and avoiding the poisons and the rats.

The next step to a healthy brain and healthy nerves is proper fuel and avoiding toxins.

Did you know that 20% of the cholesterol in your body is in your brain? When we hear cholesterol, people automatically think of heart disease and blocked arteries.

If 20% of the cholesterol found in your body is in your brain, it must have an important function in healthy people. Here's a secret, your brain and nerves require cholesterol and healthy fats to function. The medications that slow the formation of cholesterol in the rest of the body, also slow cholesterol production in the brain. Some studies link these medicines (called statins) to tingling in the hands or feet. Others even link these medicines to cases of dementia and Alzheimers

- Extra-ordinary humans work to avoid the need for medications unless absolutely necessary. As it turns out, 80 percent of the cholesterol in your body is produced by your liver when it has excess carbohydrates available. Reducing your intake of simple sugars can lower blood cholesterol levels.

However, before we go and throw out ALL the sugar you should know that the brain's preferred energy source is glucose (sugar) It uses 20-25% of the glucose in the body. So we actually need SOME sugars in our diets.

- Extra-ordinary Humans also avoid common neurotoxins in foods like MSG (Monosodium Glutamate), Artificial sweeteners like Aspartame & Sucralose, and trans fats.

These are in a class of chemicals called neurotoxins. They excite the cells and can even cause cell damage.

Now we have protected our brains from toxins and supported them with proper fats and fuels.

ADAPTATION +
RESPONDABILITY =
HEALTH

IV

Jake and I met up the next week. Grabbed our coffee and dug right in.

Doc: "So Jake, what did you find for the definition of health?"

He proudly pulled out his notebook, flipped through a few pages.

Jake: "The World Health Organization says it's

"A state of complete physical, mental and social well-being and not merely the absence of disease or infirmity"

Doc: "What does that mean?"

Jake: "Complete well being, not just ... not being sick."

Doc: "Good and what is, '*well being?*'"

Jake: "I'm not sure."

Doc: "Me neither, any other definitions?"

Jake: "Most refer back to this one, including the CDC's website."

Doc "I always found that a little unclear, ambiguous."

Jake: "How do you define health?"

Doc "What if we looked at health as your body's ability to adapt to the stressors it is exposed to?"

Jake: "Okay?"

Doc: "What are some of the stressors you can think of?"

Jake: "Getting sick with the flu or salmonella"

Doc: "Great, what are the symptoms of the flu or salmonella ."

Jake: "Feeling bad, fever, nausea."

Doc: "Great, what other kinds of stressors can you think of?"

Jake: "Um…when you are being chased?"

Doc: "True"

Jake: "How about things like being in the cold or a super hot summer day, would those also be stressors?"

Doc: "Sure"

Doc: "These are all stressors. How does your body adapt to the cold?"

Jake: "You shiver."

Doc: "Right, How does it adapt to being too hot?"

Jake: "You sweat"

Doc: "What happens if your body can't shiver or can't sweat?"

Jake: "I guess you would get sick"

Doc: "In our definition, health is your body's ability to adapt. If your body couldn't adapt it wouldn't be healthy. *Essentially, it would mean that you are already sick.*

You would be more susceptible to life threatening events like hypothermia or heat stroke."

Jake: "I guess you are right."

Doc: "So Jake, going back to the flu as a stressor is a fever bad or good?"

Jake: "Is this a trick question?"

I just smiled.

Jake: "...Bad?..." He sensed this was a risky answer

Doc: "A fever is a part of your body's adaptation response."

Jake: "How so?"

Doc: "The viruses and bacteria that are present when we are sick are multiplying. They can only reproduce within a certain temperature range. Do you know what that range is?"

Jake: "98.6 degrees plus or minus a degree or two"

Doc "Somewhere around there, when it gets a few degrees warmer, they can't reproduce. Then the rest of our immune system has less to clean up"

Jake: "So even a fever can be a sign of being healthy because we are adapting?"

Doc: "You got it."

Jake: "I like that definition of health; the body's ability to adapt."

Doc: "Me too."

Doc: "So Jake! The command center decides how to adapt and sends the message out. Where do you think adaptation could break down?"

Jake: "It could break down if that body part can't carry out the commands."

Doc: "Yup, That's the body's ability to respond. I call that respond-ability. (it's shorter) It is your body's ability to respond to the commands that the brain sends. Make sense?"

Jake: "Kind of…"

Doc: "Respond-ability requires us to be physically fit and well fed."

Working out trains our heart and lungs to be more efficient. When in danger our brain says to respond by running so we can get away from the threat.

If the brain says, 'Hey, it's hot in here!' It tells the body to sweat. If the body has water, it can respond to the command by sweating. If it is dehydrated it has low Respond-ability."

Low Respond-ability is when the body is told to respond but is not able to.

High Respond-ability is when the body is told to respond and does so quickly and efficiently.

Jake: "If people only understood that… they-"

Doc: "They would be healthy"

Jake: "Yeah"

Doc: "Maybe, but there is one huge piece that is missing. The most peculiar habit of extra-ordinary people."

Jake: "What could that be?"

Doc: "Mindset and Beliefs." I looked at my watch.

Jake: "Another cliffhanger?"

Doc: "Yup, next time. But for now.. More homework"

Jake: "Aright" He grabbed his pen.

Jake: "Ready."

Doc: "I want you to listen around or ask people why they think their health is the way it is. Bring a list of 5-6 different things they say."

Jake: "Got it."

DEFINING WHAT HEALTH IS: ADAPTATION/ RESPOND-ABILITY

The principles that exceptional people follow include the principles of Adaptation, Healing, and Strengthening.

ADAPTATION

One of the biggest signs of sickness is losing the ability to properly adapt. If you stand up and get dizzy, you have failed to adapt to changing positions.

If you run up stairs and your heart rate doesn't increase, you will pass out because your body did not adapt.

Our minds and bodies are adapting or failing to adapt all of the time:

- If your body temperature rises, the natural cooling system (sweating) helps your body to cool down (adapt)
- If your body temperature drops, the emergency heating system, shivering kicks in to warm you up. (adapt)
- When we get an infection and our adaptive resources initiate a fever. The fever raises the body temperature beyond that which the infecting virus

or bacteria can reproduce. This allows the rest of our immune responses to wipe out the invaders.

- When people get congestive heart failure (the heart muscle stretches) their body starts adapting by increasing back pressure in the arteries (caused by high blood pressure or blockage).
- If you lift weights, your body will respond to that stress by making your bones more dense. If you go to space and don't have any stress on the bones, they become thin and brittle. (Your body is adapting to the new environment and not wasting resources.)
- Adaptation occurs when we run and our heart rate goes up to pump more oxygen to our muscles.
- When we eat bad food our body's response is to make us vomit to remove the bacteria from our bodies.

When under stress, our bodies will naturally adapt for better or worse.

We see this with seemingly unrelated injuries in sports. For example a player hurts their left knee but once the knee is healed they develop a right shoulder problem from a very minor trauma. His body had adapted.

This happens because his body had started adapting to the knee injury by repositioning the shoulder. Once the knee was better, the shoulder had been weakened by its compensatory position.

With this in mind, Extra-ordinary humans don't allow injuries to stay untreated because they know that their bodies will adapt around the injury, causing more problems.

ANOTHER EXAMPLE OF ABNORMAL ADAPTATION IS CHRONIC INFLAMMATION:

Inflammation (Swelling) of the tissues is a huge part of the body's Emergency Support Network. When a tissue is cut, damaged or infected, the body starts the inflammatory response.

This signals the formation of new pain fibers in the area, laying down scar tissue and even walling off of infected areas. The inflammatory response gives us blisters and calluses. However, long term chronic inflammation leads to clogged arteries and osteoarthritis.

When a ligament (the connective tissue that holds one bone to another bone) stays inflamed, the inflamed area becomes a magnet for calcium. The calcium attaches to the ligament, over time forming a bone spur.

When an artery is inflamed, it becomes sticky to calcium and cholesterol. I recently read a heart surgeon's take on this. He noted that early in his career, he did a lot of cardiac by-pass surgeries. *(This is where they take a vein out of your leg, then remove a section of artery around the heart that has a blockage and replace that section with the vein from your leg.)* He said that back then, he saw a lot of smokers who had a localized blockage of an artery.

In recent years he has seen more people with metabolic disease where the large sections of the artery is clogged, a bypass surgery can't replace all of the damaged tissue.

Metabolic disease causes inflammation throughout the entire body.

How many times have you heard "It's just arthritis?" Or "Arthritis is normal at your age."

I refer to arthritis as a "trash bucket" diagnosis. It's where doctors throw a person's health into a trash bucket. The diagnosis covers a huge range of conditions that cause painful movement of the joints. It leads to the person taking a lot of medications for "Arthritis" to cover up the problem, but the problem still progresses.

The ligaments become inflamed and stay inflamed because of abnormal usage. If the underlying problem is identified, corrected and maintained, the bone spurs can stop growing and over time even start to reabsorb.

Inflammation leads to degeneration (an abnormal adaptation)

HEALTHY ADAPTATION:

Your brain needs balancing and stimuIlation from a variety of sources.

While the nerves in the body communicate information to the brain, a healthy brain is required to interpret all of this data and provide an appropriate response.

This is how we see this break down

There are two parts to the human nervous system and *they are opposites:*

1. One part is the **sympathetic nervous system.** This part *contracts* the smooth muscle around your arteries, raises your blood pressure, increases your heart rate, increases your breathing rate and is your basic response to physical stress. It is highly addictive. It is the excited state

2. The other part is called the **parasympathetic nervous system.** This is the part of the nervous system that *relaxes* the smooth muscles around your arteries, drops your blood pressure, decreases your heart rate, breathing rate and allows your body to rest and digest. Let's call it Rest and Digest State (R&D)

Extra-ordinary humans minimize the time they spend in the Excited state and maximizc thcir time in the parasympathetic state.

The Excited state is often referred to as the fight or flight response. It is triggered by perceived threats. Unfortunately, oftentimes your brain can't tell the difference between *real threats* and *perceived threats.* A great threat includes things that will actually kill you or your family. I am sure you could easily imagine at least 20 things that could do that. However, even just imagining and pondering on such things can trigger your sympathetic response.

If you have trained your brain to worry, then you're an expert in triggering your sympathetic response.

You can also trigger it by watching the news, getting involved in politics or thinking negatively about your future. I know people who trigger this by focusing on what they don't want. Their thought patterns and language patterns are not about things they like or who they root for. They are focused on what they don't want or who they don't like. It's like a loop of negativity and worry.

Extra-ordinary humans spend a much greater amount of their time in the Rest and Digest state.

People try all sorts of ways to get into a R&D state including drugs, alcohol, and even sex. Unfortunately these only let you temporarily escape from the sympathetic state but do not put you into parasympathetic.

How do we get into the Parasympathetic (R&D) state?
There are several ways, such as:

1. *Getting enough sleep*
2. *Avoiding the News or Politics*
3. *Moving. Particularly intentional movement like walking stimulates the R&D state*
4. *Chiropractic Adjustments*
5. *Meditation*
6. *Mindset*

RESPOND-ABILITY

While the brain nervous system decides what needs done, the body is responsible for carrying out the orders. Many of the health conditions we see being treated today are trying to change the way the body responds to the stresses that it encounters.

Extra-ordinary people train the troops before the stress occurs. One of the goals of Cross training is to stress the athlete in various ways so that they can perform in many situations.

There is a lot of research now on the health benefits of sauna therapy and ice bath therapy, because they increase the body's ability to adapt.

Average people work to decrease demands for their body to respond.

Extra-ordinary people routinely stress themselves in various ways to "train the troops" and increase their Respond-ability.

Walking, exercising, stretching, movement all stress the system.

Like we talked about earlier, they also eat better so they have "well fed and healthy troops." When the troops are called to respond, they are ready, well-trained, well-supplied, and therefore and capable of responding.

MINDSET AND BELIEFS

V

J ake and I met up at our regular time. He was more eager than ever to dive right in.

Doc: "So, where did we last leave off?"

Jake: "We were going to discuss the Peculiar mindsets and beliefs of extra-ordinary people."

Right. "What did you come up with for 'Why do people feel their health is the way it is?'"

Jake opened his notebook and started reading.

- "Look around; everyone my age…"
- "It's the food we eat"
- "I am getting old (from a 35 year old)"
- "It was the way we were raised."
- "Bad Genetics"

Doc: "That's pretty much the average mindset isn't it?"

Jake: "Yeah, they always believed it was outside of their control."

Doc: "Extra-ordinary people are peculiar in that they claim authority over their lives and decisions."

Jake: "What do you mean by that?"

Doc: "I mean if you really convince yourself to believe it's someone else's fault or outside of your control, you could have all the information in the world and nothing will change for you. You are giving them authority over your health decision."

Jake: "Some of them do sound like they're just excuses but what about genetics?"

Doc: "There are some conditions that genetics rule over like Type 1 Diabetes. Most of the time it is a genetic predisposition."

Jake: "What can we do if we have a genetic predisposition?"

Doc: "A predisposition means that it could happen, not that it *has* to happen. Families share the same genetics, but they tend to also share the same habits. They live the same lifestyle, eating the same types of foods, they may exercise or not.

The lifestyle choices both load the gun and pull the trigger on their genetics. This turns a predisposition into a condition."

Jake: "So what's the alternative?"

Doc: "A different mindset. It starts with knowing that you get to make choices and those choices have outcomes. So you make choices to gain a different mindset so you are better equipped to achieve certain outcomes. That alone is empowering."

Jake: "What kinds of choices? Like food?"

Doc: "More like we get to choose what we want, what we are working toward, how we think, and how we talk about it. They are process oriented."

I rattled off some of the Mindset's of the Extra-Ordinary to Jake-

"The people I know who are extra-ordinary do things like;
1) Speak positively about their process.
2) They look forward into the future for what they *do* want and focus on their goals and aspirations (not what they don't want)
3) They avoid negative self-talk like "I am getting old, I can't because, I used to be able to…"
4) They don't want to be average, they want to be much much better than that.
5) They avoid negative media or when they hear it, they try to keep it in perspective.
6) After they put the energy into changing something, they make the change into a positive habit.
7) They encourage other people.

8) They understand that every process takes time. So they learn to love the process and not just sprint for short term results."

Doc: "That's their mindset. Which is different from psychology."

Jake: "How so?"

Doc: "Mindset is a way of believing, psychology is the study of how things in the mind works. Understanding our psychology helps us develop principles we can use to make changes we want to make."

Jake: "Tell me about some of the psychology."

Doc: "When we look at extra-ordinary people they have different habits than average people."

Jake: "Habits are hard to change. I read that it takes 21 times of doing something to make it a habit."

Doc: "I have heard that too. But it's only partly true. Say you want to start eating better, but you dislike broccoli. If you applied this logic it would lead you to think that if you eat broccoli 21 days in a row, eating broccoli will become a habit."

Jake: "Yeah"

Doc: "I don't know about you, but eating *anything* 21 days in a row would make me HATE it, not just dislike it."

Jake: "True"

Doc: "But first, let's ask what is a habit?"

Jake: "Something that we do without thinking."

Doc: "Exactly. Our brains use more glucose (a type of sugar) than any other part of our bodies. Survival requires that it doesn't use too much energy and works efficiently. The brain has to stay alert and save enough energy in the event that something life threatening occurs.

One of its strategies is to use and establish short cuts; things which over time require less thought. As a result we establish habits; things which just become a part of our lifestyle and are incorporated into the natural rhythm of our day which in turn determine our long term outcomes."

Jake: "OK? So bad habits come from this."

Doc: Yes, but so do good habits. We usually talk about bad habits such as: increased cardiac risk, obesity, or getting caught in an emotional pattern. In contrast extra-ordinary humans leverage positive habits.

Robert Cialdini, in his book *Influence* explains psychological patterns. A habit is a psychological pattern. A stimulus causes you to go into a patterned response. He describes it like an old tape recorder, where you push the button and the tape (programed response plays)

Jake: "I never thought of it like that."

Doc: "Have you ever set up a row of dominoes then pushed them over."

Jake: "Of course."

Doc: "I like to imagine *an established habit like* a row of dominoes with a big red domino at the beginning of the line. When this big red domino gets pushed over, it starts a string of events which causes the rest of the dominos to fall over.

That is a habit; The red domino is the conditions that we either find ourselves in or we set up for ourselves that influence little decisions we make from day to day. This initiates a chain reaction of cause and effects which influence aspects of our lifestyle."

Jake: "I think I get it but how does it apply in real life?"

Doc: "Let's say we want to eat healthier. but we are tired when you get home from work and grab junk food on your way home. The red domino (being tired and hungry) cues us to do the faster and easier thing which is to grab junk food on our way home."

We want to get up in the morning and work out. What stops us?"

Jake: "The habit of hitting snooze."

Doc: "Right. What examples can you think of?"

Jake: "I plan to study for a test, practice guitar, or call mom after work , but then 11:00 rolls around and I gotta go to bed."

Doc: "Exactly! Now looking back, where did the time go?"

Jake: "Habits, like fixing dinner while scrolling on instagram or watching television."

Doc: "Right and this happens day after day, week after week and year after year. The dominoes keep falling.

Decision fatigue plays a part in it. That's when our brains are tired of making decisions. We make so many decisions every day. The Red Domino falls over and …."

Jake: "The old habit takes over."

Doc: "Uh huh. Have you ever tried making yourself do something new with 'Will Power' and reverted back to the old patterns again?"

Jake: "Of course."

Doc: "What if… we moved the red domino away from the rest? We get home and…. Boom, the big heavy domino falls and doesn't hit the rest…. Nothing happens. We stop. We look around wondering what we could be doing and easily start our new habit."

Jake: "That'd be awesome!"

Doc: "It can be unnerving at first. We are comfortable with our old habits and the set rhythms of our lives.

Shawn Achor in his book *The Happiness Advantage* he says, 'If you want to change a habit in the long term, in the beginning, you have to rely on willpower. But willpower is a finite resource and can't be relied on.'

He recommends using the 20 second rule. Make a 20 second gap between the habit cue (the red domino) and the habit."

Jake: "What do you do with those 20 seconds?"

Doc: "You have already decided what you really want to do. Then, create situations where it's easier to start your new desired habit.

Like If you want to practice the guitar, leave your guitar and music out, so you can practice easily."

For me, one red domino is staying in bed in the morning when I 'want to' work out, but where are my clothes?

I make it easier for myself by laying my clothes out the night before, when I wake up, I remember what I decided on and committed to the night before.

We get home and have to decide what to eat for dinner, but we're tired... fast food it is.

Make it easier, we prepared food for the week on Sunday. When we get home the easiest thing to do is just heat it up."

Jake: "That makes sense, It sounds easy enough."

Here's the big secret.. habits are hard to change! Once we start our automated pattern, changing directions is very difficult. What if we moved the Big Red domino so that we have time to reflect on what we are doing and what we really wanted to do.

It sounds easy, on paper. It requires 3 easy steps. 1) make a decision. 2) Define what progress (not perfection) looks like 3) move the Red domino

1) Decide your direction and destination

"If we don't know where we are going, any path will get us there." Let's get some clarity on where we want to go.

Write down where you are going. What do you want to achieve? What relationships do you want to invest in? What outcomes do you really want? What is your next step forward?

2) Define what progress, not perfection looks like

Define what progress looks like. What that looks like for you today and a year from now. What would a daily workout or walk do for you?

A weekly call to your mom, taking a class to improve your knowledge of a subject?

How will you feel about yourself 12 months from now, 3 years from now for doing this?

3) Identify what habits interfere with what you want and find what triggers that habit for you (The Red Domino) and move the red domino.

Once you identify your Red Domino, create a 20 second barrier.

And plan how you will use that 20 seconds to start your new habit pattern.

One of the really cool things about our brains is we can decide what things mean to us. When we do something, we get to decide what that means. When something happens, we get to decide **how we take it.**

Someone cut you off in traffic, does that mean that they hate you and did it "to you" ?

Or are they super stressed and having a bad day?

Was it about you, or about them?

They are gone on down the road, what do you want that to mean to you the rest of your day?

When people tell stories about their past it is called History. It should be spelled His-Story, or Her-Story because our brains filter through and interpret the events that our 5 senses bring in.

If you want to look more into that, check out the reliability of eyewitnesses of a crime. 3 people witness the same event and have completely different stories about it.

Now we use this same process to give meaning to our habits.

Average people spend a lot of time defending their habit patterns.

The defense sounds something like this...
"I drink,
watch TV,
eat junk food,
hide in the basement
You fill in the blank
every night to unplug and relieve the stress of the day."

They have given meaning to their behavior. We defend our red dominoes.

If you want to make a change, redefine your red dominoes as old patterns. The past doesn't make you good or bad.

If you want to stop thinking like that... Stop thinking like that.

Start thinking in a more empowering way.

STEP INTO THE IDENTITY THAT YOUR NEW HABIT CREATES

Past behaviors are in the past.

The best way to start new habits, new patterns, new habits is to claim the identity that goes with it.

"Never ask if someone does Crossfit, wait 10 minutes, they will tell you, then they'll tell you again." Being a Crossfitter is a positive identity.

There is no barrier of entry, you don't have to explain your level to yourself or others. If you go to Crossfit you are a Crossfit Athlete.

If you are taking Guitar lessons, you are a guitar student or player.

On the opposite side, the things you do (or don't do) determine your identity.

Once you accept your new identity as an Extra-Ordinary Human you will naturally begin to live into it!

It starts with an easy sentence, said out loud, first to yourself, then to others.

I am an Extra-Ordinary Human.

Say it now, wherever you are.

This time, we met at the office. I set up a big flip chart for Jake.

Doc: "So Jake, we have talked for several weeks. You took a lot of notes. What do you think? What are your takeaways?"

Jake: "Let me look. There was a lot!"

Doc: "Let's start with the big ideas then. Let's write them on the flip chart."

Jake flipped through his notebook, took the blue marker and walked up to the chart.

Doc: "Let's get it all up there, then we will organize it."

Jake: "Got it."

He wrote:
"Peculiar Habits" across the top of the paper
1. They Prioritize differently
2. They act differently
3. They have a different mindset
4. They use psychology to change

Doc: "Awesome!"

Jake: "thanks"

Doc: "That's their list. Now if we were to help people who want to change from Average to Extra-Ordinary. Where would they start?"

Jake: "I knew you were going to ask me that. I think, mindset."

Doc: "Why did you choose that one to be first?"

Jake: "Unless someone believes, deep down, that their choices can make a difference, none of the rest of it matters."

Doc: "Great way to put it! What's next?"

Jake: "The understanding of different priorities. Once they believe that it's possible, they need to be able to prioritize their decisions. We all have limited time, money and attention. The priorities tell us where to spend our resources."

Doc: "Then what?"

Jake: "The priorities tell them how to act but.."

Doc: "But what?..."

Jake: "If they don't understand the psychology of change, their new habits won't last."

Doc: "Smart."

He numbered them
1. Mindset
2. Understanding priorities
3. Psychology, forming new habits
4. Acting differently

Doc: "Let's grab a new sheet of paper"

He tore off the paper and posted it on the wall behind him.

Doc: "At the top of this one write Mindset. Let's summarize Peculiar Mindsets."

Jake grabbed his marker and wrote "Peculiar Mindset" across the top.

Doc: "What are the big ideas under mindset?"

Jake started writing.
1. Believe that your choices matter
2. Find and get rid of excuses
3. Only compare yourself to what is possible, not to other people
4. Be a positive encourager
5. Enjoy the process
6. Any Process takes time
7. Positive encourager of others

Doc: "Is that a good list?"

Jake: "I think it covers it."

Doc: "Me too. Next Page"

Jake tore off the top sheet wrote

Peculiar Priorities across the top of the new paper.

Doc: "OK What are the priorities?"

Jake started writing.
1. Command Center (Neurology)
2. Supply Chain (Circulation)
3. Supply Depot (Nutrition, Water and Oxygen)

Most people have these backwards

Doc: "Great! How can we protect and provide for the command center and communication?"

He wrote:
Chiropractic Adjustments,
Movement,

Music,
and Meditation.

Doc: Nice!

Large white papers started covering the walls.

Doc: "What do we do for the supply chain?"

Jake didn't miss a beat as he wrote:
Use the system (move)
Control our state (Rest and Digest vs Excitement)
Avoid the News and Politics

Great! What's next

He smiled as he tore off the paper and stuck it on the wall
next to the others.

Supply Depot:

Eat Better:
What you eat, when you eat and how much you eat.
Avoid poisons and Rats
Too much of anything is bad.

Psychology:
Change Habits
Choose a direction
Claim our identity

Finally Jake wrote
"Act Differently"

He turned to me

"I don't have bullet points for this one. We all act on our priorities and do so through our habits."

"Exactly"

Jake"And that is WHY they are Extra-Ordinary and how they get Extra-ordinary results. Once you know how and understand why they do the things they do, it doesn't seem all that Peculiar."

Now you know HOW to make changes to become more Extra-Ordinary, you know that is possible and actually quite easy.

CONCLUSION

Jake was right, once you have the Extra-Ordinary mindset you are Free. The mindset that your choices make a difference. You realize that you have a choice. You are Free to choose to make changes or not.

Knowing the Priorities of Extra-Ordinary People, helps you make better choices of where to invest your time, money and energy for the best outcomes. Remembering that living an average life or an Extra-Ordinary life is a process you will automate as much as you can, to reach your goals. Once you know how to automate your processes by changing your habits, you are Empowered.

I am excited to hear about your successes as you live the Extra-Ordinary Life.

Jeremiah,

In elementary school he had been on a special education plan called an IEP. In high school he graduated off of his IEP. They put him directly into college level courses

During the meeting, his mom heard the IEP teacher ask Jeremiah about how the chiropractic adjustment helped him? He said. "I can focus better on a chiropractic adjustment than on any of the meds I have ever been given."

In another meeting, Jeremiah and his mom were at a parent teacher conference when he was a junior in high school.

The teacher started by saying. "If I had a whole class full of Jeremiah's, my class would be perfect." Bonnie cried. When she told me, I cried too.

Jeremiah's parents had a winning mindset for him. They believed that his life could be better. They knew he could do better in school and she worked tirelessly to get him help, to bring him for appointments, and hold him accountable for his behaviors.

Average mindset could have just blamed his early life experiences and accepted low expectations for him. She believed in him and kept sharing her mindset for him.

He graduated high school and took some college classes. Today, he is an amazing young man who is following in his fathers footsteps, working at Ford Motor Company.

He still works out regularly, gets his chiropractic adjustments and eats relatively well.

We are all very proud of him and the man he has become.

Made in the USA
Middletown, DE
28 July 2023